I0416737

LOW

CHOLESTEROL

FOOD LIST

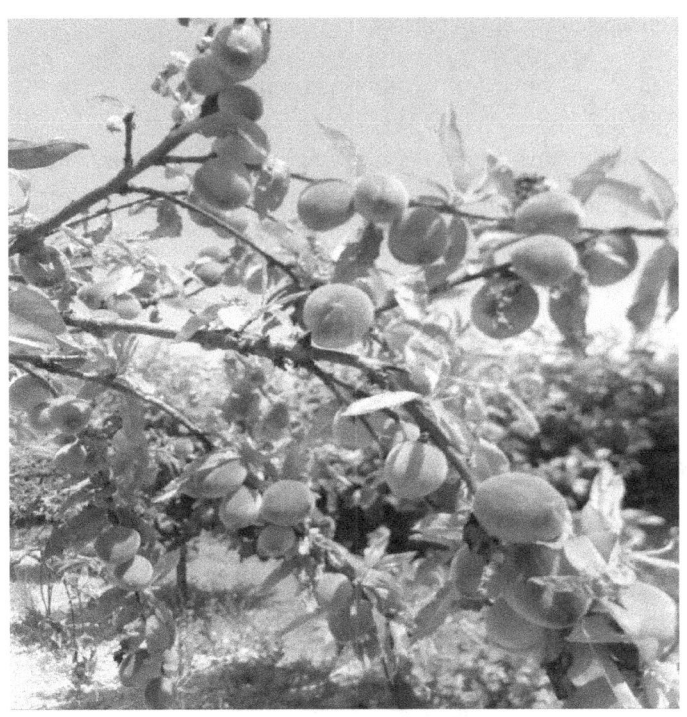

LORENE PEACHEY

TO GAIN ACCESS TO MORE BOOK BY THE AUTHOR SCAN THE QR CODE

TABLE OF CONTENTS

INTRODUCTION

In the quiet corridors of culinary exploration and nutritional wonders, I, Lorene Peachey, have dedicated my life to unraveling the secrets of a world where health meets taste, where wholesome living intertwines with culinary indulgence. For over two and a half decades, I've delved into the heart of dietary science, navigating the labyrinth of ingredients to create a symphony of flavors that not only tantalize the taste buds but also champion the cause of heart health. Welcome to my world, a realm where every bite is a step towards wellness, and every recipe is a celebration of life.

As a seasoned nutritionist, my journey began with a simple yet profound question: Can food truly be a healer, a remedy for the ailments that plague our modern lives? This question propelled me into a realm of endless possibilities, a quest to discover the alchemy of ingredients that would not just nourish the body but also rejuvenate the spirit.

Picture this – a bustling kitchen filled with the aroma of spices, the sizzle of vegetables meeting a hot pan, and the gentle hum of contentment. That's where my love affair with low-cholesterol foods started. It wasn't just a job; it was a passion, an exploration of the boundless potential that lay within the ingredients we often take for granted.

But why low cholesterol? Ah, my friend, that's the question that carries the weight of not just years of research but also the hopes of countless hearts yearning for a healthier beat. Imagine your heart as the conductor of the symphony of life, orchestrating the flow of vitality to every nook and cranny of your being. Now, think of high cholesterol as a discordant note, threatening to disrupt the harmony.

In my journey, I've witnessed the consequences of neglecting the dietary needs of our hearts. I've seen the struggle, the silent battles waged against the silent killer – high cholesterol. What starts as a seemingly harmless indulgence in rich, decadent foods can morph into a crescendo of health issues – hypertension, heart disease, and a compromised quality of life.

Let me ask you, dear reader, have you ever paused to consider the silent conversations your body engages in every time you make a food choice? Do you feel the heartbeat of your decisions echoing through the corridors of your health? The choices we make in the kitchen are not just about flavor and sustenance; they are about crafting a narrative of well-being, a story of vitality that unfolds with every meal.

As I stand on the precipice of my culinary odyssey, I am not just a nutritionist; I am a storyteller, spinning tales of nourishment, resilience, and the triumph of a heart that beats with purpose. The canvas I paint upon is your plate, and the colors I choose are the vibrant hues of fruits, vegetables, whole grains, and lean proteins – the building blocks of a low-cholesterol diet.

Let me share a secret with you – eating healthy is not a chore; it's an act of self-love. Each bite is an affirmation, a pledge to honor the sanctity of your body. The benefits are not just physical; they transcend the realms of emotion and well-being. How does it feel to know that every morsel you savor is a step towards a healthier, more vibrant you?

Can you imagine the sensation of boundless energy coursing through your veins, the buoyancy of a heart unburdened by the weight of excessive cholesterol? It's not just about living longer; it's about living better, savoring the richness of life in its purest form.

Now, let's shift our gaze to the other side of the coin, the consequences of turning a blind eye to the whispers of our health. Picture a life where every heartbeat carries the burden of excess cholesterol, where the arteries are clogged with the residue of indulgence. It's a life filled with doctor's visits, medications, and the constant fear that every bite might be a step closer to a health crisis.

Do you feel the weight of those consequences settling on your shoulders? The toll it takes on your relationships, your work, and most importantly, your relationship with yourself? It's a heavy burden to carry, my friend, and the choice to unburden yourself lies in the choices you make when you stand at the crossroads of the kitchen.

But let's not dwell on the shadows when there's a banquet of light awaiting us. Let me paint a picture of the advantages, the sheer brilliance of adopting a low-cholesterol food list into your daily life. Imagine waking up with a spring in your step, feeling the vitality surge through your veins like a river of life itself.

Consider the joy of savoring meals that not only dance on your taste buds but also nurture your body, infusing it with the nutrients it craves. Envision the empowerment that comes with knowing that every bite is a conscious step towards a healthier, heartier you.

In my extensive research, I've crafted a low-cholesterol food list that transcends the mundane. It's not about deprivation; it's about abundance. It's about exploring the myriad possibilities that reside within the realm of wholesome ingredients. The symphony I've composed isn't just for the health-conscious; it's for anyone who believes that every meal is an opportunity for transformation.

The benefits of embracing this low-cholesterol journey go beyond the physical. It's about the emotional resonance, the joy of reclaiming control over your well-being. It's about saying, "Yes, I choose health. Yes, I choose a vibrant life. Yes, I choose me."

As you embark on this culinary adventure with me, let me assure you that this isn't just a list of recipes; it's a manifesto of self-love, a declaration that your health is worth savoring. The danger of neglecting your heart's needs is real, but so is the promise of a healthier, happier tomorrow.

So, my dear friend, are you ready to flip the narrative? Are you ready to savor the flavors of a life well-lived? As we embark on this journey together, let the aroma of possibility fill your kitchen, let the colors of health paint your plate, and let the symphony of a heart in harmony be the soundtrack of your well-being.

Welcome to the world of low-cholesterol delights, where every recipe is a love letter to your heart, and every meal is a celebration of vitality. Together, let's savor the richness of life, one delicious bite at a time.

Contact the Author

Thank you for reading my book! I would love to hear from you, whether you have feedback, questions, or just want to share your thoughts. Your feedback means a lot to me and helps me improve as a writer.

Please don't hesitate to reach out to me through

lorenepeachey@gmail.com

I look forward to connecting with my readers and appreciate your support in this literary journey. Your thoughts and comments are valuable to me.

CHAPTER 1

UNDERSTANDING CHOLESTEROL

Cholesterol is a fatty, wax-like substance found in every cell of the body and is crucial for various physiological functions. It plays a vital role in building cell membranes, producing hormones, and aiding in the digestion of fat. Cholesterol is transported in the blood in two main types: low-density lipoprotein (LDL) and high-density lipoprotein (HDL).

- **LDL Cholesterol (Low-Density Lipoprotein):** Often referred to as "bad" cholesterol, LDL carries cholesterol from the liver to cells. When there's an excess, it can build up in the arteries, forming plaques that can narrow and block blood vessels.

- **HDL Cholesterol (High-Density Lipoprotein):** Known as "good" cholesterol, HDL helps remove excess cholesterol from the bloodstream, transporting it back to the liver for elimination. Higher levels of HDL are associated with a lower risk of cardiovascular disease.

Understanding cholesterol levels and their balance is crucial for maintaining heart health. Elevated levels of LDL cholesterol and low levels of HDL cholesterol can contribute to atherosclerosis, a condition where arteries become hardened and narrowed, increasing the risk of heart disease and stroke.

Importance of a Low Cholesterol Diet

Adopting a low cholesterol diet is a fundamental step in managing and preventing cardiovascular diseases. A diet that is high in saturated and trans fats, commonly found in processed foods and certain animal products, can elevate LDL cholesterol levels. Conversely, a diet rich in nutrient-dense, heart-healthy foods can contribute to maintaining optimal cholesterol levels.

The importance of a low cholesterol diet includes:

1. **Heart Disease Prevention:** Lowering LDL cholesterol reduces the risk of atherosclerosis and heart disease. By making mindful food choices, individuals can positively impact their cardiovascular health.

2. **Overall, Health Benefits:** A diet focused on low cholesterol foods is typically rich in fruits, vegetables, whole grains, and lean proteins. This not only supports heart health but also provides essential nutrients for overall well-being.

3. **Weight Management:** Adopting a low cholesterol diet often involves consuming foods that are lower in calories and saturated fats. This can contribute to weight management and, subsequently, reduce the risk of obesity-related health issues.

4. **Lifestyle Modification:** Incorporating a low cholesterol diet is part of a broader lifestyle approach to heart health. Coupled with regular exercise and other healthy habits, it can significantly improve one's cardiovascular profile.

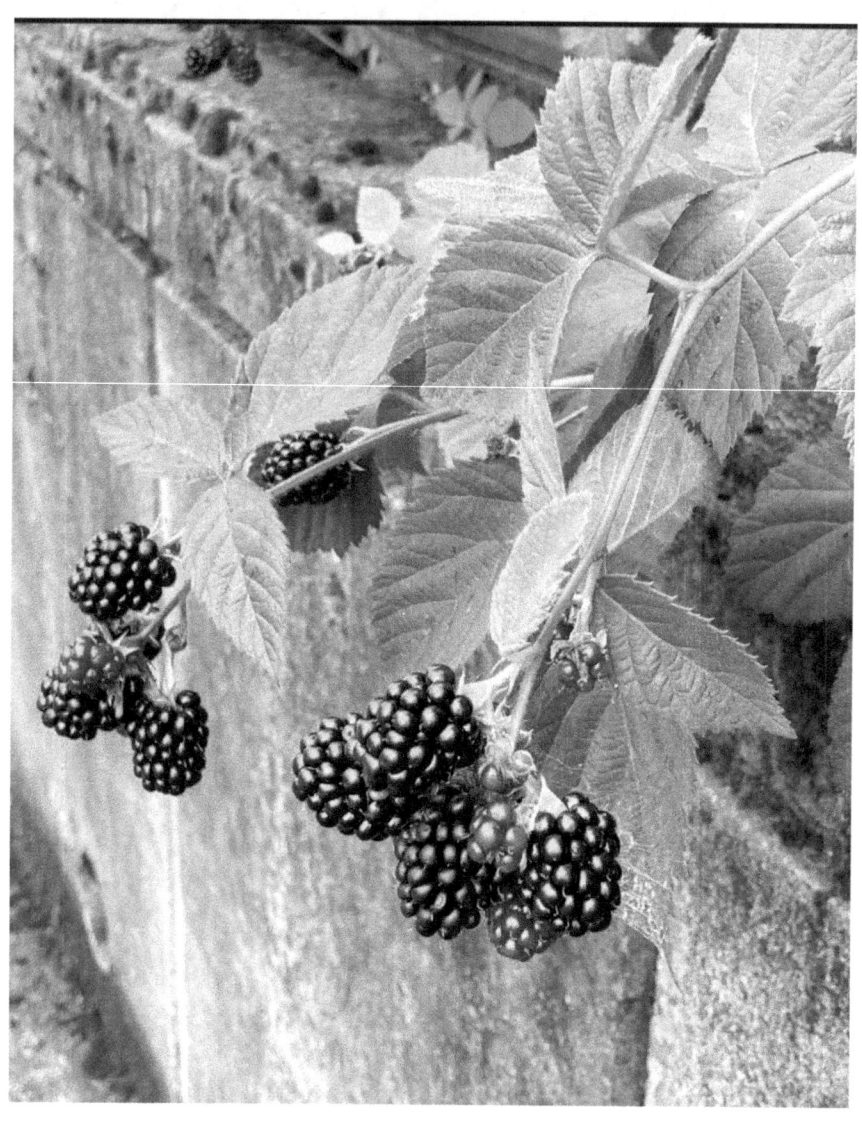

CHAPTER 2

BASICS OF A LOW

CHOLESTEROL DIET

A low cholesterol diet is a dietary approach aimed at managing cholesterol levels in the body, particularly to reduce the risk of cardiovascular diseases. Understanding the basics of this diet involves considering the types of fats consumed, making choices that promote heart health, and adopting habits that contribute to overall well-being.

What is Considered Low Cholesterol?

Cholesterol levels are typically measured in milligrams per deciliter (mg/dL) of blood. A desirable total cholesterol level is generally considered to be less than 200 mg/dL. However, it's essential to look beyond the total cholesterol number and consider the levels of LDL (low-density lipoprotein) and HDL (high-density lipoprotein) cholesterol.

- **Low LDL Cholesterol:** A healthy range for LDL cholesterol is usually below 100 mg/dL. Lower levels are associated with a reduced risk of atherosclerosis and heart disease.

- **Higher HDL Cholesterol:** For HDL cholesterol, higher levels are considered beneficial. HDL levels above 60 mg/dL are often associated with a lower risk of heart disease.

Understanding these values and working towards achieving and maintaining them through dietary choices is a fundamental aspect of a low cholesterol diet.

Dietary Guidelines for Managing Cholesterol

1. **Choose Heart-Healthy Fats:** Opt for unsaturated fats found in olive oil, avocados, nuts, and seeds. Replace saturated fats (found in red meat and full-fat dairy products) and trans fats (often present in processed foods) with healthier alternatives.

2. **Increase Fiber Intake:** Foods high in soluble fiber, such as oats, beans, fruits, and vegetables, can help lower LDL cholesterol levels. Aim for a well-balanced diet with plenty of fiber-rich foods.

3. **Select Lean Proteins:** Choose lean sources of protein, including fish, poultry without skin, legumes, and plant-based proteins. Limit red meat intake and opt for healthier protein alternatives.

4. **Incorporate Omega-3 Fatty Acids:** Include fatty fish like salmon, mackerel, and trout in your diet. These fish are rich in omega-3 fatty acids, which have been shown to support heart health.

5. **Watch Cholesterol-Rich Foods:** While dietary cholesterol doesn't impact blood cholesterol as much as saturated and trans fats, it's still advisable to moderate the intake of cholesterol-rich foods like organ meats and shellfish.

6. **Limit Processed and Fried Foods:** Processed and fried foods often contain unhealthy fats that can contribute to elevated cholesterol levels. Choose cooking methods like baking, grilling, or steaming instead.

Role of Exercise in Cholesterol Management

Regular physical activity is a crucial component of managing cholesterol levels and promoting cardiovascular health. Exercise helps raise HDL cholesterol (the "good" cholesterol) and can lower LDL cholesterol. Aim for at least 150 minutes of moderate-intensity aerobic exercise per week, along with strength training exercises at least twice a week. Incorporating physical activity into your routine complements the benefits of a low cholesterol diet, contributing to a holistic approach to heart health.

CHAPTER 3

LOW-CHOLESTEROL FRUITS

1. **Berries (e.g., Blueberries, Strawberries, Raspberries):**

   - Nutritional Information (per 1 cup):

     - Calories: 50-80

     - Fiber: 3-9 grams

     - Vitamin C: 50-100% of the Daily Value (DV)

     - Antioxidants: Anthocyanins, Quercetin

2. **Apples:**

   - Nutritional Information (medium-sized):

     - Calories: 95

     - Fiber: 4 grams

     - Vitamin C: 14% DV

     - Antioxidants: Quercetin

3. **Pears:**

   - Nutritional Information (medium-sized):

     - Calories: 100

     - Fiber: 6 grams

     - Vitamin C: 7% DV

     - Antioxidants: Flavonoids

4. **Bananas:**

   - Nutritional Information (medium-sized):

     - Calories: 105

     - Fiber: 3 grams

     - Vitamin C: 14% DV

     - Potassium: 422 mg

5. **Kiwi:**

   - Nutritional Information (medium-sized):

     - Calories: 50

     - Fiber: 2.5 grams

     - Vitamin C: 71% DV

     - Vitamin K: 38% DV

6. **Oranges:**

   - Nutritional Information (medium-sized):

     - Calories: 62

     - Fiber: 3 grams

     - Vitamin C: 85% DV

     - Folate: 10% DV

7. **Grapes:**

   - Nutritional Information (1 cup):

     - Calories: 104

     - Fiber: 1.4 grams

     - Vitamin C: 6% DV

     - Antioxidants: Resveratrol

8. **Avocado:**

   - Nutritional Information (half):

     - Calories: 120

     - Fiber: 7 grams

     - Monounsaturated Fat: 10 grams

     - Potassium: 345 mg

9. **Peaches:**

- Nutritional Information (medium-sized):

  - Calories: 59

  - Fiber: 2.3 grams

  - Vitamin C: 10% DV

  - Vitamin A: 10% DV

10. **Plums:**

- Nutritional Information (2 medium-sized):

  - Calories: 70

  - Fiber: 2 grams

  - Vitamin C: 16% DV

  - Vitamin K: 6% DV

CHAPTER 4

LOW-CHOLESTEROL VEGETABLES

1. **Spinach:**

   - Nutritional Information (1 cup, cooked):

     - Calories: 41

     - Fiber: 4.3 grams

     - Vitamin A: 377% of the Daily Value (DV)

     - Vitamin K: 1110% DV

2. **Broccoli:**

   - Nutritional Information (1 cup, chopped, raw):

     - Calories: 31

     - Fiber: 2.4 grams

     - Vitamin C: 135% DV

     - Vitamin K: 116% DV

3. **Kale:**

   - Nutritional Information (1 cup, chopped):

     - Calories: 34

     - Fiber: 2.6 grams

     - Vitamin A: 206% DV

     - Vitamin K: 684% DV

4. **Carrots:**

   - Nutritional Information (1 medium-sized):

     - Calories: 25

     - Fiber: 3 grams

     - Vitamin A: 428% DV

     - Vitamin K: 10% DV

5. **Cauliflower:**

   - Nutritional Information (1 cup, chopped, raw):

     - Calories: 27

     - Fiber: 2.5 grams

     - Vitamin C: 77% DV

     - Vitamin K: 20% DV

6. **Bell Peppers (Red, Green, or Yellow):**

- Nutritional Information (1 cup, sliced):

  - Calories: 46

  - Fiber: 3.6 grams

  - Vitamin C: 317% DV

  - Vitamin A: 93% DV

7. **Zucchini:**

- Nutritional Information (1 cup, sliced):

  - Calories: 20

  - Fiber: 1 gram

  - Vitamin C: 21% DV

  - Vitamin K: 7% DV

8. **Brussels Sprouts:**

- Nutritional Information (1 cup, cooked):

  - Calories: 56

  - Fiber: 4 grams

  - Vitamin C: 129% DV

  - Vitamin K: 219% DV

9. **Asparagus:**

- Nutritional Information (1 cup, cooked):

  - Calories: 40

  - Fiber: 4 grams

  - Vitamin A: 20% DV

  - Vitamin K: 57% DV

10. **Cabbage:**

- Nutritional Information (1 cup, chopped, raw):

  - Calories: 22

  - Fiber: 2.2 grams

  - Vitamin C: 37% DV

  - Vitamin K: 85% DV

CHAPTER 5

LOW-CHOLESTEROL WHOLE GRAINS

1. **Oats:**

   - Nutritional Information (1 cup, cooked):

     - Calories: 147

     - Fiber: 4 grams

     - Protein: 6 grams

     - Magnesium: 13% of the Daily Value (DV)

2. **Quinoa:**

   - Nutritional Information (1 cup, cooked):

     - Calories: 222

     - Fiber: 5 grams

     - Protein: 8 grams

     - Iron: 15% DV

3. **Brown Rice:**

   - Nutritional Information (1 cup, cooked):

     - Calories: 215

     - Fiber: 3.5 grams

     - Protein: 5 grams

     - Magnesium: 21% DV

4. **Barley:**

   - Nutritional Information (1 cup, cooked):

     - Calories: 193

     - Fiber: 6 grams

     - Protein: 4 grams

     - Iron: 10% DV

5. **Buckwheat:**

   - Nutritional Information (1 cup, cooked):

     - Calories: 155

     - Fiber: 5 grams

     - Protein: 6 grams

     - Iron: 12% DV

6. **Millet:**

   - Nutritional Information (1 cup, cooked):

     - Calories: 207

     - Fiber: 2.3 grams

     - Protein: 6 grams

     - Magnesium: 19% DV

7. **Farro:**

   - Nutritional Information (1 cup, cooked):

     - Calories: 220

     - Fiber: 7 grams

     - Protein: 8 grams

     - Iron: 8% DV

8. **Whole Wheat:**

   - Nutritional Information (1 cup flour, whole wheat):

     - Calories: 407

     - Fiber: 16 grams

     - Protein: 16 grams

     - Iron: 24% DV

9. **Amaranth:**

- Nutritional Information (1 cup, cooked):

  - Calories: 251

  - Fiber: 9 grams

  - Protein: 9 grams

  - Calcium: 12% DV

10. **Wild Rice:**

- Nutritional Information (1 cup, cooked):

  - Calories: 166

  - Fiber: 3 grams

  - Protein: 7 grams

  - Magnesium: 10% DV

CHAPTER 6

LOW-CHOLESTEROL LEAN PROTEINS

1. **Chicken Breast (Skinless, Grilled):**

   - Nutritional Information (3 ounces, cooked):

     - Calories: 165

     - Protein: 31 grams

     - Total Fat: 3.6 grams

     - Saturated Fat: 1 gram

2. **Turkey (Ground, 93% Lean, Cooked):**

   - Nutritional Information (3 ounces, cooked):

     - Calories: 176

     - Protein: 22 grams

     - Total Fat: 10 grams

     - Saturated Fat: 3 grams

3. **Fish (Salmon, Baked or Grilled):**

   - Nutritional Information (3 ounces, cooked):

     - Calories: 206

     - Protein: 22 grams

     - Total Fat: 13 grams

     - Omega-3 Fatty Acids: 1.5 grams

4. **Tofu:**

   - Nutritional Information (1/2 cup, firm):

     - Calories: 94

     - Protein: 10 grams

     - Total Fat: 6 grams

     - Iron: 15% DV

5. **Beans (Black Beans, Cooked):**

   - Nutritional Information (1 cup, cooked):

     - Calories: 227

     - Protein: 15 grams

     - Total Fat: 1 gram

     - Fiber: 15 grams

6. **Lentils:**

   - Nutritional Information (1 cup, cooked):

     - Calories: 230

     - Protein: 18 grams

     - Total Fat: 1 gram

     - Fiber: 16 grams

7. **Egg Whites:**

   - Nutritional Information (3 large egg whites):

     - Calories: 51

     - Protein: 11 grams

     - Total Fat: 0 grams

     - Cholesterol: 0 mg

8. **Greek Yogurt (Non-fat):**

   - Nutritional Information (1 cup):

     - Calories: 100

     - Protein: 17 grams

     - Total Fat: 0 grams

     - Calcium: 23% DV

9. **Cottage Cheese (Low-fat):**

- Nutritional Information (1/2 cup):

    - Calories: 81

    - Protein: 14 grams

    - Total Fat: 1 gram

    - Calcium: 7% DV

10. **Shrimp (Grilled or Steamed):**

- Nutritional Information (3 ounces, cooked):

    - Calories: 84

    - Protein: 18 grams

    - Total Fat: 1.5 grams

    - Cholesterol: 180 mg

CHAPTER 7

LOW-CHOLESTEROL HEALTHY FATS

1. **Avocado:**

   - Nutritional Information (1/2 avocado):

     - Calories: 120

     - Total Fat: 10.5 grams

     - Monounsaturated Fat: 7 grams

     - Fiber: 5 grams

2. **Olive Oil:**

   - Nutritional Information (1 tablespoon):

     - Calories: 120

     - Total Fat: 14 grams

     - Monounsaturated Fat: 10 grams

     - Polyunsaturated Fat: 1.5 grams

3. **Nuts (Almonds):**

- Nutritional Information (1 ounce, about 23 almonds):

  - Calories: 160

  - Total Fat: 14 grams

  - Monounsaturated Fat: 9 grams

  - Protein: 6 grams

4. **Chia Seeds:**

- Nutritional Information (1 ounce):

  - Calories: 138

  - Total Fat: 9 grams

  - Omega-3 Fatty Acids: 4.9 grams

  - Fiber: 10 grams

5. **Walnuts:**

- Nutritional Information (1 ounce):

  - Calories: 185

  - Total Fat: 18 grams

  - Omega-3 Fatty Acids: 2.5 grams

  - Protein: 4 grams

6. **Flaxseeds:**

  - Nutritional Information (1 tablespoon, ground):

    - Calories: 37

    - Total Fat: 3 grams

    - Omega-3 Fatty Acids: 1.6 grams

    - Fiber: 2 grams

7. **Coconut Oil:**

  - Nutritional Information (1 tablespoon):

    - Calories: 120

    - Total Fat: 14 grams

    - Saturated Fat: 12 grams

8. **Dark Chocolate (70-85% Cocoa):**

  - Nutritional Information (1 ounce):

    - Calories: 170

    - Total Fat: 12 grams

    - Monounsaturated Fat: 7 grams

9. **Fatty Fish (Salmon):**

- Nutritional Information (3 ounces, cooked):

  - Calories: 206

  - Total Fat: 13 grams

  - Omega-3 Fatty Acids: 2.3 grams

  - Protein: 22 grams

10. **Sunflower Seeds:**

- Nutritional Information (1 ounce):

  - Calories: 165

  - Total Fat: 14 grams

  - Monounsaturated Fat: 4 grams

  - Protein: 6 grams

CHAPTER 8

FOODS TO AVOID IN A LOW

CHOLESTEROL DIET

1. **Processed Meats (e.g., Sausages, Hot Dogs):**

   - Nutritional Information (1 hot dog):

     - Calories: Approximately 150-200

     - Total Fat: 13-16 grams

     - Saturated Fat: 5-6 grams

     - Cholesterol: 30-40 mg

2. **Fried Foods (e.g., French Fries, Fried Chicken):**

   - Nutritional Information (1 serving of French fries):

     - Calories: Approximately 365

     - Total Fat: 17 grams

     - Saturated Fat: 3 grams

     - Trans Fat: 0 grams

3. **Fast Food Burgers:**

- Nutritional Information (1 standard fast food burger):

  - Calories: Approximately 250-300

  - Total Fat: 12-20 grams

  - Saturated Fat: 4-8 grams

  - Cholesterol: 30-50 mg

4. **Commercial Baked Goods (e.g., Pastries, Doughnuts):**

- Nutritional Information (1 glazed doughnut):

  - Calories: Approximately 190

  - Total Fat: 12 grams

  - Saturated Fat: 6 grams

  - Trans Fat: 0.5 grams

5. **Full-Fat Dairy Products (e.g., Whole Milk, Regular Cheese):**

   - Nutritional Information (1 cup of whole milk):

     - Calories: 150

     - Total Fat: 8 grams

     - Saturated Fat: 5 grams

     - Cholesterol: 24 mg

6. **Processed Snack Foods (e.g., Potato Chips, Crackers):**

   - Nutritional Information (1 ounce of potato chips):

     - Calories: Approximately 150

     - Total Fat: 10 grams

     - Saturated Fat: 3 grams

7. **Margarine (Trans Fat-containing):**

   - Nutritional Information (1 tablespoon of stick margarine):

     - Calories: 100

     - Total Fat: 11 grams

     - Trans Fat: 3 grams

8. **Excessive Red Meat (e.g., Beef, Lamb):**

- Nutritional Information (3 ounces of cooked beef):

  - Calories: Approximately 213

  - Total Fat: 14 grams

  - Saturated Fat: 6 grams

  - Cholesterol: 76 mg

9. **Shellfish High in Cholesterol (e.g., Shrimp, Lobster):**

- Nutritional Information (3 ounces of cooked shrimp):

  - Calories: Approximately 84

  - Total Fat: 1.5 grams

  - Cholesterol: 129 mg

10. **Packaged Convenience Foods (e.g., Frozen Meals):**

- Nutritional Information (1 serving of a frozen meal):

  - Varies widely; often high in sodium, saturated fats, and cholesterol.

CONCLUSION

As we reach the final chapter of our culinary adventure, I find my heart brimming with gratitude and anticipation. Your journey into the world of low-cholesterol delights has been more than a compilation of recipes; it has been a shared exploration of well-being, an odyssey of flavors that resonate with the heartbeat of life itself.

In these pages, we've woven a tapestry of wholesome ingredients, transforming each meal into a symphony of nourishment. Together, we've embraced the notion that food is not just sustenance; it is an expression of self-love, a conscious choice to honor the temple that is your body. I hope these recipes have not just tantalized your taste buds but have also resonated with the rhythm of your heart, inspiring you to cherish the vitality that courses through your veins.

The benefits of adopting a low-cholesterol lifestyle are profound, extending beyond the realms of physical health. It's about reclaiming control over your well-being, experiencing the buoyancy of a heart unburdened by excess cholesterol. It's about waking up each day with a renewed sense of vigor, knowing that every choice you make in the kitchen is a testament to your commitment to a vibrant life.

But our journey doesn't end here; it's merely a pause before the next chapter. As you embark on these recipes, I encourage you to listen to the whispers of your body, to savor each bite not just for its flavor but for the vitality it imparts. Celebrate the victories, no matter how small, and relish the joy of nurturing yourself from the inside out.

Your feedback is a crucial note in the symphony we've created together. I would be honored to hear your thoughts, your experiences, and the emotions that these recipes have stirred within you. Did you discover a new favorite dish that resonated with your palate? Have you felt the transformative power of embracing a low-cholesterol lifestyle?

Your insights can spark conversations, inspire others on similar journeys, and add depth to the collective narrative of wellness. Share your stories, your challenges, and your triumphs. Let this be a community where we uplift each other, where the joy of healthy living is a shared anthem.

As you embark on the practical application of these recipes, remember that the kitchen is your canvas, and the ingredients are your palette. Feel free to experiment, to infuse these recipes with your personal touch, and to make them a reflection of your unique taste and preferences.

So, my fellow traveler in the realm of heart-healthy living, let this conclusion be a prelude to many more chapters of discovery and delight. May your journey be filled with flavor, your heart with vitality, and your spirit with the joy of savoring life in all its richness.

BONUS CHAPTER 1

HEALTHY LOW CHOLESTEROL

RECIPES

Grilled Lemon Herb Chicken

Cooking Time: 20 minutes

Servings: 4

Ingredients:

- 4 boneless, skinless chicken breasts

- 2 tablespoons olive oil

- 2 cloves garlic, minced

- 1 lemon (juice and zest)

- 1 teaspoon dried oregano

- Salt and pepper to taste

Instructions:

1. Preheat grill to medium-high heat.

2. In a bowl, mix olive oil, minced garlic, lemon juice, lemon zest, oregano, salt, and pepper.

3. Coat chicken breasts with the marinade and let sit for 10 minutes.

4. Grill chicken for 8-10 minutes per side or until fully cooked.

5. Serve with your favorite side dishes.

Nutritional Information: Calories: 280, Protein: 30g, Fat: 14g, Carbohydrates: 5g, Fiber: 1g

Quinoa Salad with Vegetables

Cooking Time: 25 minutes

Servings: 6

Ingredients:

- 1 cup quinoa, rinsed

- 2 cups water

- 1 cucumber, diced

- 1 bell pepper, chopped

- 1 cup cherry tomatoes, halved

- 1/4 cup red onion, finely chopped

- 3 tablespoons olive oil

- 2 tablespoons balsamic vinegar

- Salt and pepper to taste

Instructions:

1. Cook quinoa according to package instructions.

2. In a large bowl, combine cooked quinoa, cucumber, bell pepper, cherry tomatoes, and red onion.

3. In a small bowl, whisk together olive oil, balsamic vinegar, salt, and pepper.

4. Pour dressing over the quinoa mixture and toss to combine.

5. Refrigerate before serving.

Nutritional Information: Calories: 220, Protein: 6g, Fat: 10g, Carbohydrates: 28g, Fiber: 4g

Baked Lemon Garlic Salmon

Cooking Time: 15 minutes

Servings: 2

Ingredients:

- 2 salmon fillets
- 2 tablespoons olive oil
- 2 cloves garlic, minced
- 1 lemon (juice and zest)
- 1 teaspoon dried dill

Instructions:

1. Preheat oven to 400°F (200°C).

2. Place salmon fillets on a baking sheet lined with parchment paper.

3. In a bowl, mix olive oil, minced garlic, lemon juice, lemon zest, dried dill, salt, and pepper.

4. Brush the salmon with the mixture.

5. Bake for 12-15 minutes or until the salmon flakes easily with a fork.

Nutritional Information: Calories: 350, Protein: 24g, Fat: 25g, Carbohydrates: 2g, Fiber: 0g

Vegetable Stir-Fry with Tofu

Cooking Time: 15 minutes

Servings: 4

Ingredients:

- 1 block firm tofu, cubed

- 2 cups broccoli florets

- 1 bell pepper, sliced

- 1 carrot, julienned

- 2 tablespoons soy sauce

- 1 tablespoon sesame oil

- 1 tablespoon ginger, minced

- 2 cloves garlic, minced

Instructions:

1. Heat sesame oil in a wok or skillet over medium heat.

2. Add tofu cubes and stir-fry until golden brown.

3. Add ginger and garlic, followed by broccoli, bell pepper, and carrot.

4. Stir-fry for 5-7 minutes until vegetables are tender.

5. Pour soy sauce over the stir-fry, toss, and cook for an additional 2 minutes.

6. Serve over brown rice or quinoa.

Nutritional Information: Calories: 250, Protein: 18g, Fat: 15g, Carbohydrates: 14g, Fiber: 4g

Chickpea and Spinach Curry

Cooking Time: 30 minutes

Servings: 6

Ingredients:

- 2 cans chickpeas, drained and rinsed

- 1 onion, finely chopped

- 2 tomatoes, diced

- 3 cups spinach

- 1 can coconut milk

- 2 tablespoons curry powder

- 1 tablespoon olive oil

- Salt and pepper to taste

Instructions:

1. In a large pot, sauté chopped onion in olive oil until golden.

2. Add curry powder, tomatoes, chickpeas, and cook for 5 minutes.

3. Pour in coconut milk, bring to a simmer, and let it cook for 15 minutes.

4. Stir in spinach and cook until wilted.

5. Season with salt and pepper.

6. Serve over brown rice.

Nutritional Information: Calories: 320, Protein: 12g, Fat: 15g, Carbohydrates: 40g, Fiber: 10g

Mango and Black Bean Salad

Cooking Time: 15 minutes

Servings: 4

Ingredients:

- 2 cups black beans, cooked

- 2 ripe mangoes, diced

- 1 red onion, finely chopped

- 1 red bell pepper, diced

- 1/4 cup cilantro, chopped

- 2 tablespoons lime juice

- 1 tablespoon olive oil

- Salt and pepper to taste

Instructions:

1. In a large bowl, combine black beans, diced mangoes, red onion, red bell pepper, and cilantro.

2. In a small bowl, whisk together lime juice, olive oil, salt, and pepper.

3. Pour the dressing over the salad and toss gently.

4. Refrigerate before serving.

Nutritional Information: Calories: 240, Protein: 8g, Fat: 4g, Carbohydrates: 45g, Fiber: 11g

Lemon Herb Quinoa with Roasted Vegetables

Cooking Time: 25 minutes

Servings: 4

Ingredients:

- 1 cup quinoa, rinsed

- 2 cups water

- 1 zucchini, sliced

- 1 yellow squash, sliced

- 1 red onion, sliced

- 1 tablespoon olive oil

- 1 lemon (juice and zest)

- 2 teaspoons dried mixed herbs

- Salt and pepper to taste

Instructions:

1. Preheat oven to 400°F (200°C).

2. In a baking dish, toss zucchini, yellow squash, and red onion with olive oil, dried herbs, salt, and pepper.

3. Roast for 20 minutes, stirring occasionally.

4. Meanwhile, cook quinoa according to package instructions.

5. Fluff quinoa with a fork, and stir in lemon juice and zest.

6. Serve roasted vegetables over a bed of lemon herb quinoa.

Nutritional Information: Calories: 290, Protein: 8g, Fat: 8g, Carbohydrates: 48g, Fiber: 6g

Lentil and Vegetable Soup

Cooking Time: 45 minutes

Servings: 6

Ingredients:

- 1 cup dried green lentils, rinsed

- 1 onion, chopped

- 2 carrots, diced

- 2 celery stalks, chopped

- 3 cloves garlic, minced

- 1 can diced tomatoes

- 6 cups vegetable broth

- 1 teaspoon cumin

- 1 teaspoon paprika

- Salt and pepper to taste

Instructions:

1. In a large pot, sauté onions, carrots, and celery until softened.

2. Add garlic, cumin, and paprika; cook for 2 minutes.

3. Add lentils, diced tomatoes, and vegetable broth. Bring to a boil.

4. Reduce heat, cover, and simmer for 30-35 minutes or until lentils are tender.

5. Season with salt and pepper before serving.

Nutritional Information: Calories: 220, Protein: 14g, Fat: 1g, Carbohydrates: 40g, Fiber: 15g

Cauliflower and Chickpea Curry

Cooking Time: 30 minutes

Servings: 4

Ingredients:

- 1 cauliflower, cut into florets

- 1 can chickpeas, drained and rinsed

- 1 onion, finely chopped

- 2 tomatoes, diced

- 1 can coconut milk

- 2 tablespoons curry powder

- 1 tablespoon olive oil

- Salt and pepper to taste

Instructions:

1. In a large pan, sauté chopped onion in olive oil until translucent.

2. Add curry powder, cauliflower, chickpeas, and cook for 5 minutes.

3. Pour in coconut milk and diced tomatoes. Simmer for 20 minutes.

4. Season with salt and pepper.

5. Serve over brown rice.

Nutritional Information: Calories: 320, Protein: 12g, Fat: 18g, Carbohydrates: 35g, Fiber: 10g

Salmon and Asparagus Foil Packets

Cooking Time: 25 minutes

Servings: 4

Ingredients:

- 4 salmon fillets
- 1 bunch asparagus, trimmed
- 4 tablespoons olive oil
- 4 cloves garlic, minced
- 1 lemon, sliced
- Fresh dill for garnish

Instructions:

1. Preheat oven to 400°F (200°C).
2. Place each salmon fillet on a piece of foil.
3. Arrange asparagus around the salmon.
4. Drizzle olive oil over salmon and asparagus, sprinkle with minced garlic, and season with salt and pepper.
5. Place lemon slices on top and seal the foil packets.
6. Bake for 15-20 minutes or until salmon is cooked through.
7. Garnish with fresh dill before serving.

Nutritional Information: Calories: 350, Protein: 30g, Fat: 22g, Carbohydrates: 8g, Fiber: 3g

IF YOU WANT MORE RECIPES, YOU CAN CHECK OUT OTHER BOOKS BY THE AUTHOR

GLUTEN-FREE COOKBOOK FOR SENIORS

GLUTEN-FREE COOKBOOK FOR VEGAN

TYPE 2 DIABETES & MEAL PLAN COOKBOOK FOR

WOMEN

GLUTEN-FREE COOKBOOK FOR BEGINNERS

TO GET ACCESS TO MORE BOOKS BY THE AUTHOR SCAN THE QR CODE

BONUS CHAPTER 2

21 DAY MEAL PLAN

Day	Breakfast	Lunch	Dinner	Snack
1	Oatmeal with Berries	Grilled Chicken Salad	Baked Salmon with Quinoa	Greek Yogurt with Almonds
2	Whole Wheat Toast with Avocado	Lentil Soup with Vegetables	Vegetable Stir-Fry with Tofu	Fresh Fruit Salad
3	Scrambled Egg Whites with Spinach	Quinoa Salad with Chickpeas	Lemon Herb Chicken with Broccoli	Carrot Sticks with Hummus
4	Smoothie with Banana and Spinach	Brown Rice and Black Bean Bowl	Baked Cod with Sweet Potato	Greek Yogurt Parfait

5	Greek Yogurt with Granola	Grilled Vegetable Wrap	Chickpea and Spinach Curry	Handful of Walnuts
6	Whole Grain Pancakes with Berries	Turkey and Avocado Wrap	Baked Lemon Garlic Chicken	Apple Slices with Peanut Butter
7	Chia Seed Pudding with Mango	Quinoa and Vegetable Stir-Fry	Lentil and Vegetable Soup	Orange Segments
8	Almond Butter Toast with Banana	Salmon and Asparagus Foil Packets	Cauliflower and Chickpea Curry	Yogurt with Berries
9	Vegetable Omelette	Tofu and Vegetable Stir-Fry	Grilled Shrimp Salad	Mixed Nuts
10	Overnight Oats with Almond Milk	Black Bean and Corn Salad	Baked Tilapia with Quinoa	Fresh Fruit Smoothie

11	Avocado and Tomato Toast	Mediterranean Quinoa Bowl	Chicken and Vegetable Skewers	Celery Sticks with Hummus
12	Berry Smoothie Bowl	Lentil and Kale Salad	Baked Zucchini Boats	Cottage Cheese with Pineapple
13	Scrambled Tofu with Spinach	Whole Grain Wrap with Hummus	Baked Chicken with Roasted Veggies	Sliced Cucumber with Guacamole
14	Whole Grain Waffles with Strawberries	Quinoa and Black Bean Soup	Grilled Salmon with Asparagus	Trail Mix
15	Greek Yogurt Parfait	Chickpea Salad	Vegetable and Tofu Curry	Apple Slices with Almond Butter

16	Banana Walnut Muffins	Vegetable and Lentil Stew	Baked Cod with Lemon Herb Quinoa	Yogurt with Chia Seeds
17	Spinach and Feta Omelette	Turkey and Quinoa Stuffed Peppers	Grilled Shrimp with Brown Rice	Mixed Berries
18	Peanut Butter Banana Smoothie	Brown Rice and Vegetable Stir-Fry	Baked Chicken with Sweet Potato	Carrot and Celery Sticks
19	Blueberry Pancakes with Maple Syrup	Quinoa Salad with Avocado	Lemon Herb Tofu with Quinoa	Cottage Cheese with Berries
20	Acai Bowl with Granola	Mediterranean Chickpea Wrap	Baked Salmon with Roasted Broccoli	Handful of Almonds

21	Whole Wheat Bagel with Smoked Salmon	Vegetable and Bean Burrito Bowl	Grilled Veggie and Tofu Skewers	Fresh Fruit Salad